Food Regeneration Guide
Blood Group O Diabetic

ISBN 978-1-312-25897-6

MANUEL RAMONI... NEURO-THERAPIST

Worse Foods (*Blood Bundles, Sick and Aged*). ____ *Wheat, Milk or Cow Cheese, Pork, Delicatessen, Coffee, Melon, Tangerine, Orange, Fried Foods, Peanuts, Cauliflower, White Sugar*____

FOOD ACCORDING TO YOUR BLOOD GROUP.

BLOOD GROUP "O DIABETIC" - THE HUNTER.

What you will learn in the following pages will change your life and that of your loved ones forever and in such a precise and safe way that in a few weeks they will feel the changes in their body in such a radical and different way, that They will feel and will be younger, stronger, more vigorous, full of energy, vitality and most importantly ... Full of great **health and that when any viral or bacterial disease wants to enter their body, they will hardly feel a breakdown since** their immune system and "**ALKALINITY**" (This I will show you later) will be so strong that it will be almost impossible for them to ever get sick again (this if they keep their new culture of eating and living that I will teach them for life) and consequently take them to live the 100-year-old average.

Dr. Peter D`adamo, a deeply scientific researcher and pioneer in the field of food according to blood groups, has managed to compile through many scientific studies in different cultures and around many countries in the world. The way and way of classifying food according to the type of blood of human beings.

He managed to bring as much food as possible to the laboratory on his tour around the world and took each food and looked at it through the microscope with a blood sample of the different types that there are (4), type "O" - "A" - "B" and "AB" and managed to observe very carefully what was happening.

He managed to see that by placing the different types of food in the different types of blood, that these presented totally different characteristics from each other, that is; A) That there was a group of foods that made the blood more fluid, light and thin. B) A second group made absolutely no changes to it. C) While a third group surprisingly had clumping of the blood, that is, it made it thick and even coagulated.

So I manage to divide the food very intelligently and amazingly into three groups.

1- The foods that make the blood more fluid and less viscous or thick, making it feed (Carrying oxygen) in a very important way to all the cells of the body, passing through the thinnest capillaries of the body, nourishing, regenerating them and rejuvenating cell tissue in an extremely vital way for the body. As well as at the same time making the minute volume of the heart the most suitable for the body, thus reducing the overload that the heart needs when the blood is thick and very intoxicated... And he called them **VERY BENEFICIAL FOODS.**

2- A second group of foods that did not present or give any change in blood behavior that called them **NEUTRAL FOODS.**

3- And a third group of foods in which he noticed that in a very important way they presented clumping of the blood, making it more viscous and thick and thus hindering its function to the point that it was the main cause of premature cellular aging and called: **HARMFUL FOODS, NOT ADVISABLE OR "POISON" FOOD.** Therefore it determined after deep studies that each blood group has its indispensable food pattern and different from each other, that is, the foods that can be beneficial for a certain blood group... It is totally harmful to others.

1) **VERY BENEFICIAL: Rejuvenate, Slim, Regenerate, Regulate Cardiac Minute Volume And Extend Life.**

2) **NEUTRAL:** They feed but do not regenerate, nor do anything that group 1 does.

3) **NOT ADVISABLE:** They fatten, agglutinate (Thicken) the blood, poison the body, overload the heart, age and degenerate the cellular system.

Below I am going to expose you after many years of study and research on my part, as I have managed to summarize in broad terms the foods according to each blood group.

This I achieved thanks to GOD in tens of thousands of patients that I have seen in more than 39 years of consultation and follow-up, which with a lot of work and diligence I carried out in the deep study of each food in each blood group. Therefore, each region, country and its customs are of utmost importance.

For example, in the case of Venezuela there is the custom of the so-called pre-cooked flour or "bread flour", which has been consumed in large proportions in Venezuelan households for more than 66 years, and I realized that the sub generations following the continuous consumption of certain foods that are in principle of the group of harmful, the body adapts to the same for living and converts food HARMFUL food NEUTROS, with low toxicity, depending on the degree of generations that have crossed.

Other examples would be: Mexico, Chile (Spicy), Panamá, The Fritters, Brazil, La Feijoada (Black beans), Colombia the potatoes, Spain, Wine, etc.

Another thing that I learned unequivocally through so many years of monitoring, practice and study, is that; There are industrialized "foods" on the market that they sell to consumers in order to lose weight by substituting some of the main meals for a shake, which among other things, poorly combining, refined and industrialized carbohydrates with processed proteins (highly harmful combination, (Which we will talk about on the alkalinity life - acidification and death) In the Complete Guide to Healthy Longevity ...

That it "loses weight" but "dries" them at the same time, since the loss of collagen is progressive, and worst of all is that after the patient having spent fortunes on these "foods" they gain weight again unless they follow the diet regimen. "Products", something that will never happen with The Aliments According to its Blood Group.

There are basically three different types of protein shakes depending on the source from which those proteins are obtained, which may well be from whey (Poison for group O), egg white or soy (Poison for other groups) . The consumer does not have the slightest idea of how their body is poisoned (Acidifying it) with these drinks that keep them "full" but that far from nourishing the immune system, what is sinking it in an ending that always ends up leading to the query.

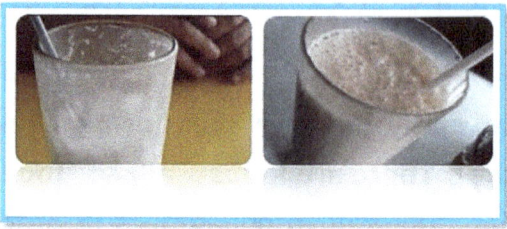

Scientific researchers at the University of California, San Francisco studied 9,000 women and found that those who consumed these products were about four times more likely to have hip fractures, among other things, than those who did not consume these "foods."

An unbalanced diet (Since it is the same "food" for everyone equally... "And no one is the same as another", especially in your blood group) "high in proteins, such as those from shakes, will directly contribute to having fragile bones or osteoporosis among other serious conditions that you will have in the medium or short term, more likely in some than others, depending on your vitality and blood group.

"Eating these artificial and highly harmful" foods "is like smoking and saying ... "It doesn't hurt me"

Keep in mind that according to the different food cultures that I will indicate for each blood group in particular, there are also people who are "secretory" and "non-secretory".

SECRETORS. A person is secretory, regardless of their blood group. It is when the antigens of your blood group are present both in your blood and in your body fluids and secretions, such as saliva, intestinal mucus or respiratory cavities, semen, etc.

NO SECRETARIES. A non-secretor, it does not secrete antigen from its group in its fluids but only in its blood.

Many metabolic characteristics such as carbohydrate intolerance or immune susceptibilities are genetically linked to the non-secretory subtype. A certain disadvantage is supposed compared to the "secretors", since these, when secreting the antigen from their blood group in their saliva and the intestinal mucus, have "extra" protection against certain microorganisms and lectins of some foods.

Another additional advantage of secretors is that they are able to maintain a more stable ecosystem of bifid intestinal bacteria suitable for their group. Most of these bifid bacteria use their blood group as the preferred food source, and since secretors have a higher blood volume in the intestinal mucus, their bacteria benefit from a more constant supply of food.

Approximately 80% of the world population are "secretaries". While 20% are Non-Secretaries. Therefore, it is important to repeat that the following list of foods according to your blood group has been adapted to correct these disagreements when shopping at the supermarket. And something of which I will be very emphatic... DO NOT PUT ANY FOOD OUT OF YOUR BLOOD GROUP IN THE CART WHEN MAKING THE MARKET for you.

With this new culture of eating, you will be able to eat whatever you want and as many times as you want to eat, as long as it is in the range of foods indicated according to your blood group, such as those that are advisable and neutral, but never the "poisons". You will not only lose weight quickly and progressively, but a date will come when you will not lose weight anymore since at that moment you will have reached your ideal natural weight and can continue eating as many times as you want during the day and <u>NOT</u> You will never gain more weight in your life and if you are a thin person, then not only will you feel better, but you will soon be in your necessary size and according to your age, but with a full immune system on top and prepared to fight any attack exogenous...

> It is for this and other reasons that you will see in the course of the content of this Guide that I have successfully managed to eradicate diseases from a sick body and cure patients ranging from simple obesity to cancer of any kind and thanks to GOD. In more than 45 years of experience and unless it is due to natural causes, I HAVE NEVER LOST A PATIENT...

BLOOD TYPE "O DIABÉTIC" – THE HONTER.

All people in group O carry in their blood a genetic memory of strength, endurance, boldness, intuition, self-confidence and innate optimism. Who has inherited the leadership and success trend that thrives on good health and optimism.

Meat consumer. Strong digestive tract. Very active immune system. Intolerant to environmental and dietary adaptations. Respond better to stress with intense physical activity. It requires an efficient metabolism to stay slim and energetic. It has fluid blood that resists clotting as it lacks some clotting factors.

Your digestive tract transforms fats and proteins into ketones, which are used in place of sugars to keep glucose levels stable. **Dairy and cereals are not beneficial to you** like the other blood groups because your digestive system is not fully adapted to them. The success of your diet depends on your consumption of lean (fat-free) meats, poultry, and chemical-free fish.

The main factor for weight gain is the gluten found in wheat germ and all wheat flour products, whether whole or not, because they act on your body creating the opposite state of ketosis, as lectins in Gluten inhibits your insulin metabolism, interfering with the efficient use of calories. **Corn, to a much lesser degree** (especially in Venezuela).

There are other factors that contribute to your weight gain. Certain beans and legumes, especially lentils **and beans**, contain lectins that are deposited in your muscle tissues, making them less "gifted" for physical activity, since your muscles need to be in a state of slight metabolic acidity, thus using up calories. More quickly.

The third factor is related to thyroid regulation, since people of blood group O have a **tendency to low levels of thyroid hormone**. Hypothyroidism occurs because type 0 does not usually make enough iodine. **Symptoms include weight gain, fluid retention, muscle weakness, and fatigue**.

It appeared more or less 40,000 years ago. Their digestive system is adapted to a diet rich in animal proteins and the vegetables they can find. Dairy products and cereals were not yet part of our diet since Agriculture and livestock will not appear until about 30,000 years later.

1- **Meat consumer.**
2- **It has a resistant digestive tract.**
3- **Very active immune system.**
4- **Intolerant to environmental and dietary adaptations.**
5- **Respond better to stress with intense physical activity.**
6- **Requires an efficient metabolism to stay slim and energetic.**
7- **Group O is the oldest blood group.**
8- **It developed when humans were hunters.**
9- **People with this group easily digest animal proteins and fats, but have difficulties**

assimilating dairy, grains, rye, semolina and cereals.

10- **44% of Caucasians and 48% of blacks have the "O" blood type, which is why it is called universal.**

11- **In these people the introduction of animal proteins in their diet with an adequate proportion of animal fats is essential to avoid fatigue and mental and organic depression.**

12- **Exercise is also important for your physical and mental well-being.**

People in group O can digest and metabolize meats very efficiently and quickly because they are often high in stomach acid. However, you should try to balance your meat proteins with the appropriate fruits and vegetables to avoid excessive acidification that can cause ulcers or irritation of the stomach lining.

Next I will indicate the list of foods for group **"O" DIABETICS** updated and compiled with studies of many years of strategic follow-up for each blood group. That they will make them lose overweight and diseases of any kind of which they are knowingly possessed or that these diseases are in you in full development and you still do not know it.

PEOPLE WHO WANT TO LOWER THEIR WEIGHT AND VOLUME.

They have to suspend, sweets, beers, flours and all carbohydrates during the treatment to lose weight, whether they are **Very Beneficial** or Neutral. Because they interfere with the purification of the body. And after they have reached their ideal weight they will be able to eat these foods as long as they are in the beneficial foods.

Next I will indicate the list of foods for group O updated and compiled with studies of many years of strategic follow-up for each blood group. That will make them lose overweight and diseases of any kind of which they are possessors with knowledge or that these diseases are in full development and you do not know it yet.

It is of utmost importance due to the change of name of foods according to the region, the country or the culture; that when they get the name of a food in the lists that I indicate below and they do not know it. **Search the Internet with the name of the food and its synonym.** Then **with the name of the food in question, look** in the part **of Google images** and thus you can recognize the food.

Formula for the "Diabetic 0"

ELIMINATE ALL KINDS OF SUGAR FROM YOUR DIET, YOU CAN SWEET WITH ESTEVIA BUT LITTLE AND IN A MODERATE WAY.

It is very important to make the three main meals and the three snacks since your metabolism is highly energy consuming ... You should never miss in your snacks (in addition to what you want to eat within your allowed meals) vegetable salads with salmon, broccoli and green tea.

Beneficial Meats	25%
Neutral Meats	10%
Beneficial Vegetables	25%
Neutral Vegetables	10%
Beneficial Tea	10%
Beneficial or Neutral Carbohydrates	10%
Rest of the Neutral and Beneficial Foods	10%

Practice this formula the best you can and you will see in a short time how it reduces your disease until it disappears completely from your body in cases of type 2 and type 3 diabetes. While in type 1 diabetes or insulin dependent mellitus you will gradually notice how their diabetes is reduced until in many cases the habit of taking insulin is eliminated, in others until the dependence on insulin is drastically reduced. While in the most chronic cases it will reduce at least between 40 and 60% of insulin dependence, achieving in all cases profoundly improving the person's quality of life.

In diabetic groups, it is practically the same formula as non-diabetic groups. The difference is that the diabetic groups have to eliminate their sugar and excess carbohydrates to bring them to a safe cure in cases of type 2 and 3 diabetes, while in cases of type 1 diabetes or insulin-dependent in many cases insulin it will be eliminated by installing the new culture that I present to you in this Guide, (But above all in the indications and recommendations that you will find in the Healthy Longevity Guide) and in other cases not only will the amount of insulin that is injected daily be considerably reduced, but also it will greatly improve your quality of life.

MEATS.

Very Beneficial: **Beef, Ram (sheep, sheep), Heart, Lamb (sheep, goat, goat), Buffalo, Liver, Veal (beef), Venison.**

Neutral: **Ostrich, Rabbit, Pheasant, Hen, Duck, Turkey, Partridge, Chicken.**

Not Advisable: Pork, Quail, Fried Meals, Goose, Ham, Bacon, Turtle.

FISH AND SEAFOOD.

Sea products, the second most concentrated animal protein, are more appropriate for individuals with type O blood. Fatty fish in cold waters are excellent, which favor the adhesion of platelets such as **salmon**. Fish oils are very effective in treating inflammatory bowel conditions such as colitis or Crohn's disease to which they are susceptible. **Make seafood the main component of your diet.**

Very Beneficial: Herring, Cod, Mackerel (Bonito), Bucket,, Carite, Sturgeon, Hypogloss, Horse mackerel, Sole, Smooth, Pike, Hake, Red and White Snapper, Yellow Perch and White Perch, Sunfish, Swordfish, Shad, Salmon, Salpa, Sardine, River Trout.

Neutrals : Abalones (abalone), Clam, Anchovy, Eel, Tuna, Bream (mojarra or pancho), Shrimp, Crab, Carp (river fish), Corocoro, Cataco, Catalana, Cazón, Dorado (Mahi mahi), Smelly (river smelt), Lobster, Prawn, Mussels, Grouper, Oysters, Monkfish, Sailfish, Snook, Sea Turtle, Sea Trout.

Not Advisable: Pollock (Kinglet or species of cod), Rana's Anca, Catfish, Barracuda, Caviar, Squid, Sea Snails, No Fish Vinegary, Fish of Yellow Meat of River or Lake, Octopus, Scallops, Do not Eat Smoked Fish, Salmon Eggs, not "cured" with salt.

EGGS AND DAIRY PRODUCTS.

Dairy should be restricted because it is not metabolized well. Tofu and milk are excellent high-protein alternatives.

Some people in this group may eat four to five eggs a week and small amounts of dairy, but dairy is generally a poor source of type O protein. Still, especially if you are a woman, try to take a daily calcium supplement. , since dairy is the best natural source of assimilable calcium, preferably **de-lactose-free milk**.

THERE ARE NO DAIRY OR CHEESE THAT ARE BENEFICIAL FOR THE "O DIABETIC" GROUP.

Neutral: Eggs 3 to 4 weekly (Chicken or Duck), Soy Milk, Almond Milk, Lactose-Free Milk, Mozzarella Cheese, Soy Cheese, Goat Cheese, Sheep Cheese (Feta), Butter (animal), Walnut Margarine .

Not Advisable: Camembert, Casein, Cottage, Curd, Sour Cream , Skimmed, De Bola (Edam), Emmenthal, Gruyere, Quail Egg, Goose Egg, Jarlsburg, Whole Milk, Skim Milk, Goat Milk, Coconut Milk, Cheddar, Kefir, Brie Cheeses, Cream Cheese, Munsters, Neufchatel, Parmesan, Provolone, Whey, Swiss, Ricotta, Roquefort, All varieties of Yogurt, Yogurt.

OILS AND FATS.

Group "O" reacts well to oils. They can be an important nutritional source and an aid to evacuation as long as you limit your consumption to monounsaturated oils such as **olive and flax seed**, which have positive effects on the heart and arteries and contribute to lower cholesterol in blood.

Very Beneficial: Oil of almond, oil of Nuez, oil of olive, oil of linseed (seed of flax).

Neutrals: Oil Liver Cod, Oil, Coconut Oil of sesame (sesame) oil of gooseberry, butter.

Not Recommended: Safflower Oil, Canola Oil, Sunflower Oil, Corn Oil, Peanut Oil, Evening Primrose Oil, Cotton Seed Oil, Castor Oil, Soybean Oil.

DRY FRUITS AND SEEDS.

You can find a good source of **supplemental** plant protein in some varieties of nuts and seeds, however **these foods should in no way replace protein-rich meats. They are high in fat and you should avoid them if you are trying to lose weight**. They can cause digestive problems if they are not chewed well.

Very Beneficial: Nut in General, Pumpkin Seeds, Flax Seeds.

Neutrals: Almond, Hazelnut, Cocoa, Water Chestnut, Dried Figs (no sugar), Dried Apricots (no sugar), Almond Margarine, Sesame Margarine (sesame), Smooth Walnut, Castile Nut, Pine Seeds, Seeds of Sesame.

Not Advisable: Breadfruit, Peanuts, Pistachio, Peanut Margarine, Sunflower Margarine, Chinese Mamón, Merey, Para Nut or Para Chestnut, Poppy Seed, Sunflower Seeds.

VEGETABLES.

To those belonging to blood group O, **some legumes** inhibit the metabolism of other important nutrients such as those found in meat and **reduce acidity to the muscle tissue** of this group, which they need to perform better. **This should not be confused with the acid-alkaline reaction** that occurs in your stomach. In **this case, the few very beneficial legumes are the exception.** These promote the strengthening of the digestive tract and the healing of ulcerations and should be eaten in moderation. Grains should be avoided to a minimum until your diabetic condition is cured.

Very Beneficial: Peas (petipoas, peas, peas), Bay Beans, Pinto Beans.

Neutrals: Caraota (should be eaten in moderation), Chickpeas, Soybean Germ, Cochinera Bean and Common.

Not Advisable: Grains of Any Type that are not Indicated Above, Coffee, Lentils, Common White Beans, Red Beans, Tamarind Beans.

CEREALS.

Whole wheat flour products or not. They are not tolerated by this "O" blood group and should be totally eliminated from the diet. **They contain lectins** that react with both your blood and your digestive tract and interfere with the proper assimilation of beneficial foods. **Its gluten interferes with type O metabolic processes,** thickening and clumping the blood dangerously quickly.

Do not forget that the excess of these carbohydrates, although they are necessary, decreases the body regeneration time for the diabetic if they eat them above the indicated formula.

Very Beneficial: None.

Neutrals: (in small quantities, but necessary due to carbohydrates), mainly: Brown Rice, White Rice, Amaranth, Oats, Rye, Rice Cream, Oatmeal, Corn Flour Mixed with Rice (little), Rye Flour (rye products), Spelled (it is a variety of wheat), Soybean Flour, Quinoa, Cooked Millet, Rice Bran, Buckwheat, Turanicum (Egyptian wheat).

Not Recommended: Barley, Corn Flakes, Breakfast Cereals, Cream of Wheat, Starch, Popcorn, Wheat Germ, Corn Flour, Wheat Flour, Corn Flakes, Corn, Wheat Bread or Whole Wheat Bread and none other than the neutral ones, Oat Bran, Wheat Bran (bran), Semolina, Shredded Wheat.

BREADS.

The only breads this group can eat are Hebrew breads, made with sprouted grains because the gluten lectins (in the seed coat) have been **destroyed in the germination process**. The Ezequiel and the Essene (they are obtained in some naturist houses) are nutritious and conserve many intact enzymes, they can be obtained in health food stores. Do not forget that these carbohydrates (I insist) you can eat them **YES**, but in small quantities, due to your condition, until you cure your diabetic condition.

Highly Beneficial: Bread Essene, Ezekiel bread.

Neutral: Rice Cakes, Unrefined Rice Bread, Rye Bread, Spelled Bread, Soybean Flour Bread, Millet Bread, Rye Toast.

Not Advisable: Multi Cereals, Unleavened Wheat Bread, Crumbled Wheat Bread, Hard Wheat Bread, Hyper Protein Bread, Corn Muffins, English Bread, Wheat Bread and Whole Wheat Bread, Wheat Bran Bread (bran), Pumpernickel, Wheat Bread Threads.

PASTA.

Since most pasta **is made with wheat semolina**, be careful to choose those made with buckwheat pasta, tupinambo or rice flour (in Chinese supermarkets you get rice pasta), which are better tolerated but **not essential for your diet**. You can eat these pasta, but in small quantities, maximum 1 times a week, until your diabetic condition is cured.

Very Beneficial: None.

Neutrals: Artichoke Pasta (artichoke), Basmatí Rice Pasta, Indian Pasta, Barley Pasta, Rye Pasta, Spelled Pasta.

Not Advisable: Noodles, Germinated Wheat Flour, Semolina Pasta, Wheat Semolina Pasta, Couscous, Spinach Pasta, White Flour Pasta, Oatmeal Pasta, Gluten Paste, Graham Pasta, Bulgor Wheat Pasta, Pasta Durum Wheat, Whole Wheat Pasta, Semolina.

VEGETABLES.

There is a huge amount of vegetables available to this group that **are a critical component of their diet**. Others, on the other hand, **can cause serious problems such** as some of the cruciferous family (Brussels Sprouts and Cauliflower) that **can inhibit thyroid function in type 0.**

Very Beneficial: Garlic, Garlic Porro, Chili, Kombu Seaweed, Pumpkin, Broccoli and Romaine Lettuce (rich in vitamin K), Chard, Chicory, Artichoke, Seaweed, Celery, Cardoon (tuna cardon), Onions in General, Chives, Cabbage Curly, Kohlrabi, Dandelion, Endive (endive, Brussels chicory), Spinach, Beet Leaves, Turnip in General, Potato (sweet potato), Parsnip (parsnip, white carrot), Parsley, Red Peppers, Quimbombó, Horseradish, Jerusalem artichoke.

Neutral: Green Olives (without vinegar), Agar, Peas, Watercress, Eggplant, Bamboo Shoots, Radish Sprouts, Coriander, Coriander, Zucchini, Chinese Cabbage (bok choy), Chayote, Shallots (small onion in the form of garlic), Dill, Escalonia (onion shaped tomato), Asparagus, Broad beans, Fennel, Mushrooms, Ginger, Common Lettuce, China, Yellow Turnip, Yam, Yellow Pepper, Potato, Tomato Paste, Paprika, Radish, Radicheta, Beetroot, Rutabaga (Swedish turnip), White and Colorado Cabbage, Tomato, Thyme, Yucca (little), Pods, Carrot.

Not Advisable: Black Olives, Cauliflower and Brussels Sprouts, Ocumo (otoe), Chinese Ocumo, Leek, Cucumber, Rhubarb, Zabila (no product).

FRUITS.

There are many fruits available for type O that, in addition to being an important source of fiber, vitamins and minerals, can be an **excellent alternative to breads and pasta.**

Very Beneficial: Blueberries (mirtillos), Cambur Manzano (little), Cherries, Plums (all), Guava, Fresh or Dried Figs (without sugar), Prunas (purple or purple fruits cause a more alkaline reaction, which **balances the acidity** in her digestive tract), Gala Apple.

Neutrals: Avocado (little), Elderberry, Persimmon, Cocoa, Carambola (star fruit or Chinese tamarind), Plums Raisins (not sweet), Coconut (Little), Damascus (apricot), Dates, Peaches, Raspberries, Granada, Currant (berry, blackberry), Soursop, Fig of Tuna, Kaki, Lechosa or Papaya (little), Lima, Lemon, Mamón, Mango snack (little), Blackberries, Apples in General, Peach, Nectarine (little), Pears, Pineapples (very little), Ripe plantain Parboiled (little), Grapefruit (grapefruit), Quinotos (Chinese oranges), Blackberry.

Not Advisable: Bananas (large cambur), Sugar Cane, Strawberries, Kiwi, Tangerines, Melon (high mold content), Orange (no type), Loquat, Litchi (walnut or Chinese hazelnut), Parchite, Currants (raisins), Tamarind.

FRUIT JUICES AND LIQUIDS.

Vegetable juices are preferable to fruit juices, <u>due to their alkalinity.</u> If you choose a fruit one, choose a variety that is low in sucrose and not from the factory.

Very Beneficial: Mineral Water, Spinach Juice, Spinach Juice, Cherry Juices (very alkaline), Plum Juices, Prune Juices, Guava Juice.

Neutrals: Lemon Water (water, little lemon and Stevia sugar), Celery Juices, Blueberry Juices, Damascus Juices (apricot), Lechosa Juices (little), Natural Apple Juice, Nectarine Juice (little), Juice of Tomato shucked, Grapefruit Juice, Juice carrot, lime juice, pear juice Natural.

Not Advisable: Coconut juice, Industrial Apple Juice, Cabbage Juices, Tangerine Juice, Orange Juice, Cucumber Juices, Tamarind Juice, Parchite Juice, Industrial Blackberry Juice, Grape Juices, Apple Cider, Zabila in any Presentation.

SPICES.

Very Beneficial: Red Alga and Black Alga (counteract hyperacidity), Carob, Chili Pepper, Red Elm Bark

Garlic, Turmeric, Curry, Ginger, Parsley, Cayenne Pepper.

Neutrals: Agar (seaweed gelatin), Savory, Moruno, Basil, Capers without Vinegar, Anise, Arrowroot, Saffron, Stevia Sugar, Bergamot, Cinnamon (very little), Cardamom, Chives, Cocoa, Cloves, Cumin, Coriander, Coriander, Cream of Tartar, Mushrooms, Dill, Essence of Almonds, Tarragon, Wintergreen, Gelatin, Laurel, Yeast, Marjoram, Mint, Mustard without Vinegar, Mustard Powder, Oregano, Paprika, Paprika Powder, White Peppercorns, Pepper English, Bell Pepper, Licorice Root, Radish, Rosemary, Sage, Soy Sauce, Tartar, Thyme, Cat's Claw.

Not Recommended: Vinegar Capers, Corn Starch (cornstarch), Aspartam, Starch Sugar, Refined Sugar, Fructose, Glucose, Guarana, Sugar Cane Syrup, Corn Syrup, Maple Syrup, Junípero, Molasses, Honey, Nutmeg, Ground Black Pepper, Apple Cider, Vinegar, Balsamic Vinegar, White or Red Wine Vinegar, Vanilla.

CONDIMENTS.

Very Beneficial: Basil, Saffron, Cloves, Curry, Yellow Ginger, Laurel, Parsley, Powder of the Carob Fruit.

Neutrals: Baker's Yeast, Mayonnaise without vinegar, Mustard, Homemade Seasoned Sea Salt.

Not Recommended: Corn Starch, Marinade, Cubes, Pickles or Vinegar Vegetables of all kinds, Ketchup or Tomato Sauce (**from the vinegar**), Fructose, Glucose, Fruit Jelly, Corn Syrup, Fruit Jam, Nutmeg, Pepper black.

HERBAL INFUSIONS (tea).

Very Beneficial: Fenugreek (fenugreek), Álsine (chickweed or stellar), Cayenne, Dandelion, Ginger, Hops, Mint, North American Elm, Rosehip Tea, Linden. Parsley, Rosehip and Sarsaparilla **protect the immune and digestive system.**

Neutrals: White Birch, Birdseed, Candelaria, White Oak Bark, Skullcap, Ginseng, Raspberry Leaf, Catnip, Chamomile, Marjoleto or Hawthorn, Horehound, Yarrow, Flaxseed, Sage, Elderberry, Green Tea, Thyme, Cat's Claw, Valerian, Verbena.

Not Advisable: Alfalfa, Aloe (aloe), Sesame, Burdock, Corn Beard, Shepherd's Bag, Gentian, St. John's Wort, Strawberry Leaf, Rhubarb, Sen, Black Tea, Red Clover, Horse's Claw.

DRINKS (stimulants).

Very Beneficial: Seltz Water (sparkling water), Spinach Juice.

Neutrals: Lemon Water (little lemon, water, Stevia sugar), Beer (low alcohol content), Sparkling or

Chapinized Wine, Wines (very little, no sugar), Less Hypertensive.

Not Advisable: Coffee (even if it is decaffeinated), Cola, Soft Drinks of Any Kind, Malt, <u>Distilled Liquors of No Kind</u> , Black Tea.

SUPPLEMENTS FOR THE "O DIABETIC" TYPE.

The goal is to add the missing nutrients to your diet and provide extra protection where you need it to speed up metabolism, increase blood activity, prevent inflammation, and stabilize thyroid function. **You can take 500 mg of vitamin C daily for life at breakfast**.

Vitamin D is not necessary because many foods are fortified with **vitamin D and the best source is sunlight.**

Vitamin B: Accelerates metabolic processes. **Folic acid and vitamin B-12** are beneficial for depression, hyperactivity, and attention deficit along with the Type 0 diet and an **exercise** program. **Avoid using a formula that contains yeast or wheat germ**. You can get it in **meat, liver, kidney, nuts, leafy vegetables, fish, fruit.**

Vitamin K: It is not recommended as a supplement, so it must be consumed in **liver, egg yolk, lettuce, spinach, chard.**

Calcium: You must take strong supplementation (110-600mg of elemental calcium, daily) due to the tendency of the blood group "O" to **develop arthritis and inflammatory joint processes.** You must eat protein to increase its absorption. **(Thornless sardines, salmon, broccoli, kale, walnuts).**

Iodine: To avoid weight gain, fluid retention and fatigue, it is recommended to eat **saltwater fish, shellfish, seaweed.** Do not overdo cooking since Iodine is destroyed by cooking.

Manganese: (With caution in this group O). It is necessary only for people with chronic joint conditions (especially in the knees and lower back) for short periods and under medical supervision, since the main source of this mineral is legumes and whole grains. **It is in the walnut, peas, beans, beans, pods.**

Not Advisable:

Vitamin A: Take supplements derived from fish oils IN A LITTLE AMOUNT because they reduce the fluidity of your blood. Take it from sources rich in vitamin A or beta-carotene. Fat **carrots, spinach, tomatoes, lettuce and green leafy vegetables in general, asparagus, apricot, liver.**

Vitamin E: May slow clotting. **Get it from olive oil, liver, nuts, recommended green leafy vegetables.**

Foods that Degenerate.

- **Gluten from wheat**: Interferes with the efficiency of insulin, slows the metabolic rate.
- **Corn**: It interferes with the efficiency of insulin, slows the metabolic rate.
- **Beans-beans**: They impair the use of calories.
- **Lentils**: They inhibit the proper metabolism of nutrients.
- **Cabbage, cauliflower and cabbages**: They inhibit the production of thyroid hormones.

Regenerating Foods.

- **Fish, shellfish, seaweed and iodized salt**: They contain iodine that favors the production of thyroid hormone.
- **Liver**: Source of vitamin B that favors an efficient metabolism.
- **Red meat**: Promotes efficient metabolism.
- **Spinach and broccoli**: They promote efficient metabolism.

OTHER RECOMMENDATIONS...

- **Healthy Longevity Book... How to Live 100 Years Appearing Much Less.**
- **The Cookbook... Personalized According to your Blood Group.**
- **Certified Courses for Professionals and Aspiring Therapists.**

The House of Children Foundation...
We recommend the "BOOK TO

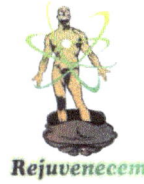

HEALTHY LONGEVITY GROUP A DIABETIC".
The goal... Live 100 years Appearing much less... Because if you can... **Bring:**

➤ How to eat and Rejuvenate according to your Blood Group.

➤ Special Exercises to Increase Health.

➤ Golden Tips that will make you lead a Much Better Life.

➤ How to eat after 45.

➤ How to Regenerate Metabolism.

- How to clean the liver, bile ducts, colon and kidneys.

- Alkalinity Life - Acids Death.

- How Emotional Conflicts Kill.

- Why We Age and How to Rejuvenate (2,023)...

- Local and Systemic Mushroom Cleaning

- 9 Foods to Have More Intense Intimate Relationships.

- The 12 Best Nutrients for Life Extension.

THE KITCHEN RECIPE FOR DIABETIC GROUP A...

It is personalized according to your blood group, where you can prepare delicacies that will rejuvenate you and in a simple way.... **Bring:**

- How to Prepare the Best Sauces.

- How to Prepare the Best Mayonnaise.

- Preparation of Smoked Bones at home.

- Prepare the best Chimichurri or Guasacaca that you have ever eaten.

- Italian Sea Salt, For Salads, Meats, Seafood, Fish and Poultry.

➤ Broths for: Meat, Seafood, Chicken, Chicken, Fish.

➤ Unrivaled Starters, Salads, Soups, Creams and Main Dishes.

➤ Yyyy of course the best Christmas dishes.

And remember that your Blessing will Help Many Needy here at La Casa De DIOS Foundation and where we will be praying for your seed to be paid in health for you and you're Family.

The Cookbook will find it at this link. www.fundaciondeterapeutas.com

COURSES.

✚ Certified Courses for Professionals and Aspiring Therapists.

Sai-Medic Institute for Scientific Research.
Attacking the Cause. Effects Disappear.
Center for Alternatives
Scientific Health Research.

Rejuveneceme

With more than 45 years of experience in hundreds of thousands of patients and using the latest advances in science, we will indicate you with simple, but powerful recommendations, how to treat the problems that afflict humanity in such a fast and palpable way, that you will believe. Find out why we get sick and age. How to quickly rejuvenate and heal...

Ownership of the Course Certified by the Institute will be delivered.

Professional Courses.

COURSE Chosen.

1- Neuro Advanced Acupuncture. Energy Systems.

2- Food to have more intense relationships.

3- How to Regenerate According to the Blood Group.

4- How to Rejuvenate.

5- Cancer If Cured.

6- Obesity ... Lose Weight Immediately.

7- How to cure type 2 diabetes in a short time.

"May GOD be our Strength"

CURRICULUM VITAE

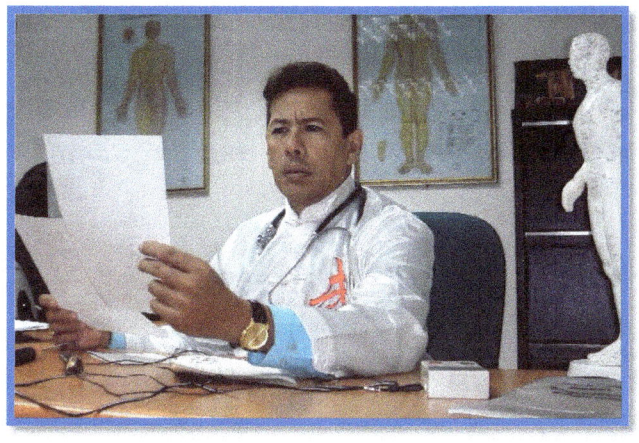

Name: M. A Ramoni

Web: fundaciondeterapeutas.com

Professional Studies:

- ENAHO (National School of Acupuncture and Homeopathy). Years 1983 to 1989.

- Studies at the Venezuelan School of Psychotronic Society. 1989 Caracas Venezuela.

- Studies of the Food Yin Yang Macrobiotic knowledge of Dr. Sakurazawa Nyoiti of Japanese origin, through Professor Omar Viera.

- Korean Acupuncture (Koryo Sooji Chim Acupuncture Mano koryo) from Master Dr. Yoo Tae W received with a Three Level program at the National School of Acupuncture and Homeopathy through Dr. Omar Viera.

➤ Studies of Dr. José Luís Padilla Corral, director of the School of MT Ch. "Neijing" Spain.

➤ Regression hypnosis INME Institute (Experimental Meta-gnomic Institute).

➤ Didactic Homeosineatry. From the Bathem Bathen school.

➤ Iridology. International Federation of Iris Diagnosis. From the Federation of Dr. Omar Viera.

➤ Maxilo-Facial anti-wrinkle treatment through the dermatron and electo-acupuncture. 2009 (I continue).

➤ Food According to the Blood Group. Research researcher James and Peter D'adamo. 2008. (I continue).

➤ Rejuvenation through the lengthening of the telomeres. 2010 (I continue).

➤ Alkalinity and acidity of cells in the development of diseases. 2010 (I continue).

➤ Master in Energy Systems.

- Master in Anesthesia by Electro Acupuncture.
- Master in Pain Therapies.
- Master in Iridology (Diagnosis by Iris).
- Neuropsychology. The New Medicine of the Future. Dr Hamer Germany.

JOBS:

- President and founder of the Scientific Research Institute of Alternative Health Medicines SAID-MEDIC.
- Director of the Said-Medic La Maracaya Medical Center clinic from 1988 to 1992.
- Director of the Said-Medic Lourdes Medical Center clinic from 1993 to 1995.
- Director of the Said-Medic Medical Center clinic Dungeon from the year 1996 to the year 2,000.
- Professor in courses for Doctors and Para-Doctors in Homeopathy - Acupuncture 1st Level - 2nd Level - 3rd Level and Energy Systems.

➤ Director of the Las Acacias Said-Medic Medical Center clinic from the year 2010 to the year 2012.

➤ Director of the Said-Medic Palmarito Medical Center clinic from year 2013 to year 2017.

➤ Director of the Said-Medic Street Páez Medical Center clinic from 2.017 to 2.023.

➤ Professor, Lecturer, International Bioenergetics Seminary - Neuro Acupuncture - Food according to the Blood Group - Why we age and how to rejuvenate - Main diseases, Neuro Psychology, among others.

WRITER OF MEDICINE BOOKS:

1- Rejuvenate, lose weight, be strong and healthy.

2- Food According to Blood Group "O".

3- Blood Group Healthy Longevity Guide A.

4- Blood Group Healthy Longevity Guide A Diabetic.

5- Blood Group Healthy Longevity Guide AB.

6- Blood Group Healthy Longevity Guide Ab Diabetic.

7- Blood Group Healthy Longevity Guide B.

8- Blood Group Healthy Longevity Guide B Diabetic.

9- Blood Group Healthy Longevity Guide O.

10- Blood Group Healthy Longevity Guide O Diabetic.

11- Food According to Blood Group "A"

12- Food According to Blood Group "B"

13- Food According to the Blood Group "AB"

14- Food According to the Diabetic Blood Group "O"

15- Food According to the Diabetic Blood Group "A"

16- Food According to the Diabetic Blood Group "B"

17- Food According to the Diabetic Blood Group "AB"

18- Blood Group Cookery Recipe "O".

19- Blood Group Cookbook "A"

20- Blood Group Cookbook "B"

21- Blood Group Cookbook "AB"

22- Cooking Recipe Group Diabetic Blood "O"

23- Cooking Recipe Group Diabetic Blood "A"

24- Cooking Recipe Diabetic Blood Group "B"

25- **Cooking Recipe** Diabetic Blood Group "AB"

26- Cancer if cured ... Educate, Alkalize and Balance.

27- Slimy Blood Syndrome ... The Cause of All Diseases.

28- How to Cure the Prostate.

29- Free yourself from Arthritis.

30- Farewell to Rheumatism.

31- Obesity ... Lose Weight Immediately and never Gain Fat again.

32- Alkalinity Life - Acidity Death.

33- Diabetes if Cured.

34- Say Goodbye to Hypertension.

35- Constipation ... Dark Future.

36- Convert your Pain into Well-being ... Legs, Lumbago, Sciatica, Spine and Cervical, among others.

37- Regenerate yourself from ACV

38- How to Eliminate Kidney and Gallstones.

39- Liver, Bile Duct, Gallbladder and colon cleansing

40- Cure Gastritis and Gastro Esophageal Reflux.

41- Say goodbye to asthma.

42- Because we grow old.

43- Tell me your Conflict ... And I will tell you that you suffer.

OTHER BOOKS:

1- CROSS POETRY. (Poetry, Updating).

2- 7 MINUTES. (Thriller, Updating).

PROFESSIONAL ASSOCIATIONS:

- Member of the WHO (World health organization number 0023 for Latin America, in alternative health medicines, through ENAHO).

- Member of the International Acupunture Association.

- College of Homeopaths and Natural Alternative Medicine Sciences.

- Venezuelan Federation of Natural Alternative Medicines N° 0024V as well as Member of the International Centers of Homeopathy and Acupuncture of: CHCMANV N° CHV002-A - INCIHOVE N° 00020 AVA 051-V.

SPECIALTIES.

1- Diagnostic Specialist.

2- Cancer if cured.

3- Neuropathies.

4- Column.

5- Cervical.

6- Some (pain) of any kind.

7- Type 2 and 3 diabetes If it is cured.

8- Type 1 diabetes (Mellitus) exponentially improves the quality of life.

9- Arthritis.

10- Rheumatism.

11- Obesity.

12- Diseases without Cause Diagnosis.

13- Migraine, Headache.

14- Digestive System.

15- ACV

16- Body, Mental and Dynamic Rejuvenation.

17- Asthma.

18- Allergies.

19- Lupus.

20- Emotional Conflicts.

21- Traumas.

22- Renal Deficiency.

23- Neurological Senile dementia, Parkinson's, Alzheimer's, Huntington.

24- Seizures.

25- Hypertension ... Among many others.

"If we eliminate the cause ... the effects are eliminated."

"The Course that Rules Nature ...

It is the Artistic Expression of *GOD*."

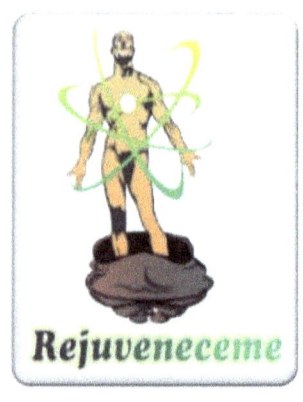

Now, reread one by one the important topics that you will find in the Healthy Longevity Guide, in relation to the new culture of rejuvenation - healing and get rid of once and forever, that damaged state that so much hinders a body healthy.

www.fundaciondeterapeutas.com   2.023.

DEDICATION...

I want to dedicate this and all the good things I have done in this world to the one who deserves it the most and that is my Heavenly Father.

Jehovah of Hosts...

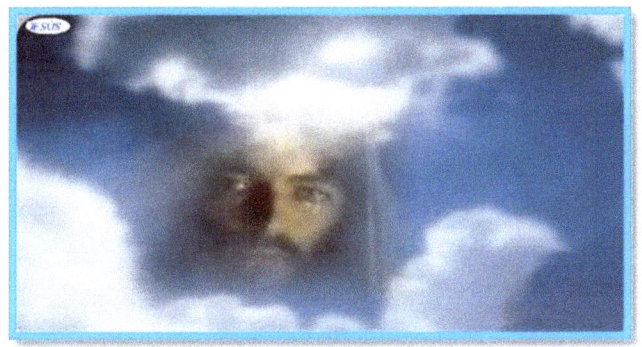

Thank you, I love you very much and... In the name of *GOD* ...I wish you the best...

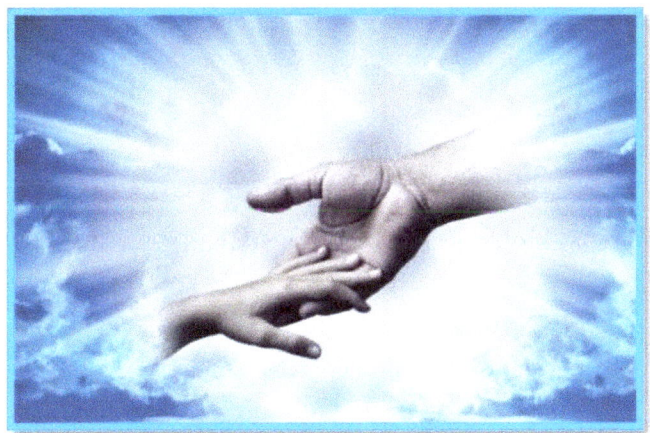

So... Never forget, that when science says... I can't anymore... *GOD* says... I start...

www.ingramcontent.com/pod-product-compliance
Lightning Source LLC
Chambersburg PA
CBHW070433180526
45158CB00017B/1189